TIPS FOR INSULIN-DEPENDENT DIABETICS

Stewart H. McLennan

CONTENTS

1   Blood Glucose Monitoring   1

2   Insulin Administration   9

3   Diet Plan   19

4   Treating Hypoglycemic Attacks 33

5   Physical Activity   40

6   Social Life   46

7   Travelling   52

8   Prescriptions   57

PREFACE

The intent of this eBook is to serve as a useful guide for all insulin-dependent Diabetics looking to improve their diabetes management and subsequently lower their HbA1c (average blood glucose level). This eBook supplements general advice you may receive from health professionals, providing detail and tips acquired from both firsthand experience and detailed scientific research. In addition, the eBook can be used as reference for everyday situations a Diabetic may find themselves in and can be referred back to whenever in doubt.

In the interest of being concise, it is assumed the reader has a baseline knowledge of diabetes i.e. terms such as 'blood glucose measurement' (a measurement of the amount of glucose in a person's blood) and 'hypo' (shorthand for a 'hypoglycemic attack') are already familiar. None the less, the eBook has been laid out and detailed in a way to help make it accessible to the majority of readers. Each Chapter ends with a bullet summary of the tips it covered, providing an 'at a glance' overview of the key takeaways.

For those Diabetics who already feel they have a good grasp over their management and simply want to make small adjustments here and there, it is recommended you skip around the contents of the book using the contents page to get to the information you desire. Please don't feel obligated to read the eBook from start to finish.

CHAPTER 1
BLOOD GLUCOSE MONITORING

Choosing a Testing Device

The most common testing device used for measuring blood glucose (BG) level is a basic finger-stick BG meter which comes with a lancet device and insertable testing strips. Over time BG meters have developed to become smaller in size, less invasive and more accurate.

It is good practice to replace your BG meter once a year. By doing so, this will help mitigate any issues such as calibration errors that may result from extensive use of the device. In addition, the BG meter market is constantly updated with technological advancements, such as smaller blood sample requirements to give readings, greater data capacity and less painful lancet devices. If you live in a country or state where you have to pay for new devices, I would recommend contacting the manufacturer of your current device and explain you've had the current device for a while and want to request a new one on warranty. In my experience most manufacturers are happy to do this free of charge.

In recent years, continuous glucose monitors (CGM), also known as 'flash' monitors, have entered the diabetes care market. This normally involves wearing a small circular patch (the sensor), which is about 1.5 inches in diameter, on the posterior of the upper arm. Most CGM sensors last for two weeks before declining in accuracy and needing to be replaced. The sensor continuously reads the users glucose level 24/7 with readings being obtained by simply holding a small BG meter or smart phone over the sensor and holding it there for a few seconds. The advantage of this is that in most cases the CGM automatically takes BG readings every five minutes and stores the data for the user to view whenever desired. This allows the user to see trend graphs of how their BG levels are behaving throughout the day, over night and on average over longer periods of time (Fig. 1). All of this is done without the user having to constantly take manual readings. Naturally, this can prove very beneficial in catching specific trends such as times of the day where you may be going too low or too high. In turn you can use the data to adjust your insulin routine accordingly.

Despite the many benefits CGM offers, it's important to note that it is not measuring BG levels directly from the blood. The CGM reads BG levels from interstitial fluid which has a lag time in terms of giving the users current BG level (Fig. 2). This lag time is approximately 10 minutes compared to the standard 'finger-stick' BG meter which only has a lag time of approximately five minutes [1, 2]. The reason for the lag in the finger-stick test is due to the time needed for BG to transport from the intravascular to the interstitial compartment of the body. It is therefore important to keep a normal BG meter on you at all times when you opt to use a CGM, as this should be used when an urgent BG reading is needed such as during a hypo and when a delay in the BG reading could be problematic. Note that, although being relatively small, the lag time for finger-stick tests varies according to the testing site. This is discussed in more detail in the 'Testing Sites' section of this chapter.

BG measurement devices give readings in either millimoles per litre (mmol/L) or milligrams per decilitre (mg/dL). A millimole is one-thousandth of mole where a mole is measured as 6x1023 molecules or atoms of a particular substance. A milligram is one-thousandth of a gram and a decilitre is one-tenth of a litre. Most devices are required to meet an accuracy standard of being within 0.8mmol/L (15mg/dL) for BG levels of less than 4.2mmol/L (75mg/dL) and within 20% for BG levels greater than or equal to 4.2mmol/L, as issued by the International Organization for Standardization [3].

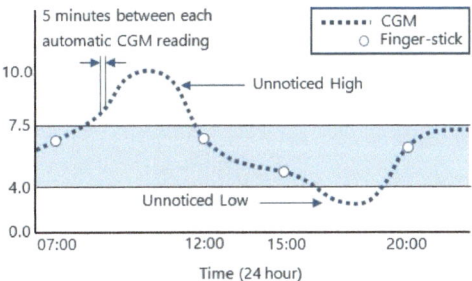

Figure 1 Example daily trend graph produced by a CGM. Note that the CGM picks up data that a finger-stick BG meter would not.

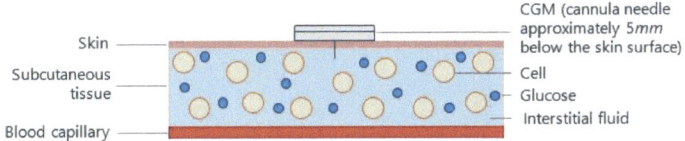

Figure 2 CGM measuring blood glucose in the interstitial fluid.

When to Test

Most health professionals recommend that at a minimum, insulin-dependent Diabetics test at the following times:

- Upon waking up
- Before meals
- Before going to sleep
- Anytime you may feel you are having a hypo
- 10-15 minutes following treatment of a hypo

Note that if the test 10-15 minutes after treating a hypo is still too low (less than 3.5-4.0mmol/L) it is recommended that the person further treats the hypo and then tests again 10-15 minutes following this. This process should be repeated until the BG levels are above 3.5-4.0mmol/L. Note that further information on treating hypos is provided in Chapter 4.

Although not necessary, and perhaps inconvenient to some, I personally like to test one hour following meals in addition to the aforementioned testing times. This allows me to see if I have correctly accounted for the carbohydrates I have eaten with my insulin administration and if I need to correct for any mistakes I may have made. More information on accounting for carbohydrates with insulin is provided in Chapter 3. It is also important to test before and after any exercise, and possibly during as well depending on the intensity, duration and type of exercise being carried out. Please refer to Chapter 5 for detailed instructions on best practice for BG testing around exercise.

As previously mentioned a CGM removes the requirement for manually testing BG levels overnight, however, I am aware many insulin-dependent Diabetics do not have access to a CGM. If this is the case, I recommend performing overnight tests for one night every one to two months using your finger-stick BG meter. This involves setting an alarm for every one to two hours throughout your normal sleeping duration and simply recording your BG levels while making sure to not correct if the level is too high. The reason for not correcting your BG level if it is too high during an overnight test (i.e. administering insulin to lower your BG) is that you want to use the obtained results (good or bad) to assess if your current insulin regime is correct. This is easier to draw conclusions from if you simply watch what is going on overnight. The following day the overnight BG readings can be analysed and appropriate adjustment can be made to you insulin regime. Of course if you pick up on a hypo during a night test, then this should be treated straight away. Having performed this many times I can appreciate how much of an inconvenience it is and have had to deal with feeling very tired the following day, however, I feel it is definitely something an insulin-dependent Diabetic should do at minimum once every 2 months due to the benefits it can have on your BG control.

Overnight hypos are a scary thought due to fact we are not lucid enough to treat the hypo when it occurs and as such they can often go un-noticed. There are a few aspects to overnight hypos that make them particularly dangerous; firstly, if you are having a severe hypo you're unlikely to be able to alert anyone for help. Secondly, if overnight hypos are a regular occurrence and going un-noticed, they can cause a Diabetic to lose their hypo awareness which in turn prevents them from noticing future hypos in their early stages. Thirdly, it is believed by number of health professionals that repeated hypos can lead to impaired cognitive function as a result of repeatedly starving the brain of glucose. I should add that the research into that final point is not as comprehensive as the other points made, however the studies that have been conducted do suggest a link with hypos and impaired cognitive function.

Testing Sites

As previously mentioned, for finger-stick tests the reading delay is dependent on the testing site being used on the body. It is recommended that in order to get the most up-to-date reading (minimum delay) one uses their fingertips as the primary testing site. The fingertips are filled with small blood capillaries that are continually flowing with blood and as such give a good indication of the exact BG level at the time of testing. This is because BG readily transports from the intravascular to the interstitial compartment in the fingertip zone. In comparison, if a person test on their forearm the BG reading will be not as up-to-date due to blood being more stagnant in the forearm zone, compared to the fingertip zone. There is no exact answer to the specific delay times by testing site, however, from my own experience I would say BG readings carry an approximate delay of five minutes for a fingertip test and 15 minutes for a forearm test.

Due to the skin damage induced by continuous pricking of the fingertips, it is recommended that the sides of the fingertips, not the centre, be used as the testing site. The reason for this is that the fingertip is packed with nerve endings which are essential for touch and feel and can become damaged upon long term testing, however, the sides of the fingertips are less sensitive and less important for touch and feel. In addition, fingertip testing should be rotated around both hands so as to not over stress one fingertip. I would also advise that the index finger and thumb tips be avoided as a testing site, the reasoning being that these are act as pincer fingers that play a major role in terms of touch sensitivity when picking things up, so it follows that it is beneficial to avoid damage to the nerve endings at these zones.

Other sites you may wish to use for testing, that provide reasonably accurate readings, are the palm of the hand and back of the hand. All of the recommended testing sites on the hands are illustrated in Figure 3.

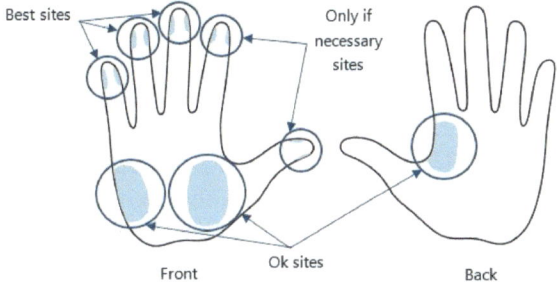

Figure 3 Standard and alternative BG testing sites.

Blood Glucose Monitoring Tips Summary

- Replace your BG meter once a year
- Always try and request new BG meters on warranty
- Use CGM to catch specific trends such as times of the day where you may be going too low or too high, and adjust your insulin regime accordingly
- Be mindful that CGM readings carry a lag time of approximately 10 minutes compared to the standard finger-stick tests which only has a lag time of approximately five minutes
- Test one hour following meals in addition to the aforementioned testing times.
- Aim to perform overnight testing one night every two-four weeks and adjust your insulin regime accordingly
- Use your fingertips as the primary testing site
- Use the sides of the fingertips for testing, not the centre
- Fingertip testing should be rotated around both hands to avoid skin damage
- Index finger and thumb tips should be avoided as a testing site.

CHAPTER 2
INSULIN ADMINISTRATION

Understanding Insulin Types and Action Times

The two most commonly used insulin types are 'rapid-acting' and 'long-acting' insulin also known as 'bolus' and 'basal' insulin, respectively. In addition to these two, a number of other types exist, all of which have varying action times. A detailed list of these insulin types along with their respective brand names is given in Table 1.

Table 1 Various action times of insulin types and their respective brand names [4].

Type	Brand Name	Onset [1]	Peak [2]	Duration [3]
Rapid-acting	Humalog NovoRapid Novolog Apidra	10 - 30 minutes	0.5 - 3 hours	3 - 6.5 hours
Long-acting	Lantus Levemir	0.8 - 2 hours	NA	12 - 24 hours
Short-acting	Regular	0.5 - 1 hours	1 - 5 hours	6 - 10 hours
Intermediate-acting	NPH	1 - 2 hours	6 - 14 hours	16 - 24 hours

[1] Length of time before insulin takes effect
[2] Length of time over which insulin is most effective
[3] Total length of time over which insulin takes effect

Sticking with the two main types, here I will explain how a better understanding of their action times and characteristics can lead to better Diabetes control. Typically, rapid-acting insulin takes 10-30 minutes post-injection to begin to take effect, depending on the brand of insulin being used [4]. The rapid-acting insulin then reaches its peak effect approximately 1.5 hours post-injection and then slowly decreases in action from here until approximately 4.5 hours post-injection where the effect becomes more or less negligible. As for long-acting insulin, this has a steady state effect for approximately 24 hours and should be injected every day at the same time (or twice a day if one is using Levemir brand insulin). While most health professionals say the effect of long-acting insulin is constant throughout the day, it actually varies somewhat depending on the time it is injected. This is illustrated in Figure 4, where it can be seen that the insulin action (level) has a slight dip towards the end of the 24 hours post-injection i.e. it is not a perfectly straight line.

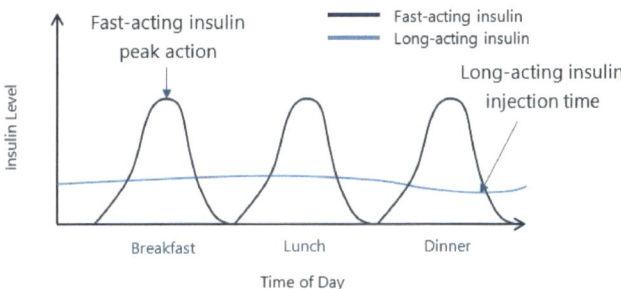

Figure 4 Graph showing comparison between mealtime insulin action time (bolus) and long-acting (basal) insulin action time.

A useful tip for anyone on a rapid-acting and long-acting insulin regime is to firstly look up graphs showing the insulin level against time for each insulin type and/or brand being used. Then, by comparing the graphs for each against one another the specific times of the day where there may be more or less insulin acting in the body than desired can be identified. For those who are more tech savvy I would recommend overlaying the action-time graphs of both rapid- and long-acting insulin on Excel to gain a clearer picture, as shown in Figure 4.

To further explain why this is a useful exercise, I will

give you a personal example. At one point in time I was using the brands NovoRapid (as my rapid-acting insulin) and Lantus (as my long-acting insulin) and while I thought my regime was correct I was still having high BG readings from 5pm to 7pm. By mapping out action-time graphs of the two insulin types, I realised the highs were caused by the drop-off in effect of the long-acting insulin at 5pm, which made sense given I injected it at 7pm every day. From realizing this I was able to simply correct the issue by taking slightly more rapid-acting insulin with my evening meal to counteract to slow-acting insulin drop-off.

Injections Areas

Administration of insulin from both insulin pens and insulin pumps for all types of insulin should be done into subcutaneous fat, which is the fat just below the skin. If you are like me and carry very little body fat, you may find that even the smallest pen needles often go straight through the subcutaneous fat and into the muscle directly below. If this is the case, a good solution is to pinch the skin at the injection site using your thumb and index finger and then injecting into the raised skin fold. This keeps the needle within the area of subcutaneous fat as shown in Figure 5.

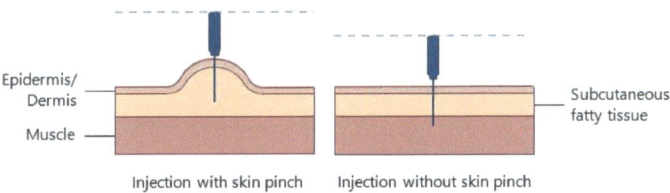

Epidermis/
Dermis

Muscle

Subcutaneous
fatty tissue

Injection with skin pinch   Injection without skin pinch

Figure 5 Schematic of insulin injection into the subcutaneous tissue (the tissue between the skin and the muscle layer below). Note that the left side illustration shows the advantage of raising the skin by pinching with the thumb and index finger.

Again from personal experience, I occasionally find when injecting that I prick a small vein below the skin surface. When this happens it causes slight bleeding and bruising, however there is no need to worry when this happens as most likely it will only be a small blood vessel close to the skin surface that has been damaged. It is very unlikely you will damage a major vessel when injecting without intentionally trying to do so as the needles are generally far too short to reach a major vessel.

Another issue I have encountered is swelling of the

skin immediately after injection in the form of a small lump at the injection site. Again there is no cause for concern when this happens as this is simply caused by some of the insulin not quite reaching the fat tissue and sitting just below or in the skin, and in most cases the insulin will quickly dissipate into the fat tissue where it is meant to be and will then act in the intended fashion.

A number of injection sites exist on the body with the most commonly used being the abdomen. An illustration of recommended injection sites is given in Figure 6. It is important to continually rotate injection sites to ensure one area is not being overused as this can lead to damage of the skin and fat tissue which in turn prevents insulin from acting effectively when subsequently injected in that area. Much like rotating across your fingers when testing your BG levels, it is good practice to rotate your injection sites.

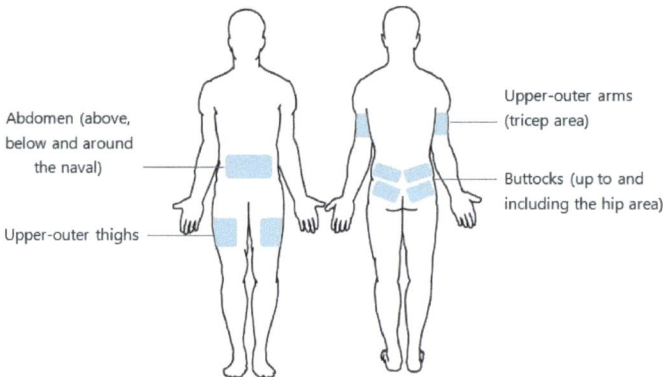

Figure 6 Recommended insulin injection sites.

When selecting injection sites, those who carry more fat on their body are at an advantage as most of the recommended sites as shown above require an adequate amount of fat tissue for insertion of the pen needle.

Conversely, for those with less fat on their body, certain areas such as the thighs and arms simply don't carry enough fat tissue to inject into. Signs that the injection site is not 'fatty' enough are when a 'nippy' or 'stingy' sensation is felt upon injecting into the site and/or the injection is causing skin lumps at the site, similar to the lumps previously mentioned. If this is the case the best areas to use, purely from a comfort standpoint, tend to be the abdomen and upper buttocks while employing the pinching technique as mentioned before.

Moving away from discussion of injection sites and considering post-injection, it is helpful to rub the injection site to get blood flowing in the area and thereby causing the insulin to act faster. As a side note, you may have had some health professionals tell you to allow insulin to warm to room temperature (25-30°C/77-86°F) prior to administering it for a quicker action time, however, personally I find this does not make any noticeable difference.

Finally, it is important to remember that most insulin products can no longer be used 28 days after opening them as the quality of the insulin reduces with time. Therefore, it is best to store insulin in the fridge at a stable temperature of approximately 4°C (39°F) to prevent freezing, which can damage the insulin [5].

Administering Using an Insulin Pump

Although most of the discussion in this chapter is focused on pen injections, it is important to also discuss insulin pumps which are being more and more commonly used. Fortunately, much of the underlying principles of insulin injection and action are the same for both pens and pumps, however, a few important differences will be highlighted here.

Firstly, most pumps only require rapid-acting insulin to be inserted into them prior to use. This is due to the pumps ability to slowly release the rapid-acting insulin it uses in small increments, normally every five minutes, which simulates the effect of slow-acting insulin meaning it is not required. Whenever the user of a pump requires rapid-acting insulin, say to cover the carbohydrates of a meal, the pump simply injects the necessary amount of fast-insulin (as programmed by the user) while the continuous slow release of insulin to simulate slow-acting requirements carries on in the background.

In my opinion, pumps carry many advantages over pen injections. The first advantage is that a pump user can fine tune their insulin requirements. Pen users can normally inject insulin in single units or half-units of insulin (IU) whereas most pumps can administer down to a range of 0.02-0.05IU. Note that one unit of insulin (1IU) is equal to 1/100th of a milliliter (ml) of insulin. This allows pump users to more accurately correct their BG levels and match their carbohydrate intake with their insulin. A second advantage is that the slow-acting insulin regime of a Diabetic can be carefully varied using the pump settings. This is done by adjusting the amount of slow-acting insulin being administered at certain times of the day which the pump will then remember to do until a future adjustment is made. To further illustrate using personal example, I require less slow-acting insulin overnight and as a pump user I am able to program my pump to give me less insulin during this time. Another 'slow-acting' advantage is that most pumps have 'temporary basal (slow-acting)' settings where the user can reduce or increase their basal insulin amount for a one-off defined period of time. This is very useful following exercise where the body requires less insulin due to the muscles being starved of glucose and during spontaneous activities such as shopping where the body also requires less insulin. More information on insulin requirements and exercise is provided in Chapter 5. A third advantage is that pumps are often more convenient for Diabetics who live busy lifestyles. The act of simply pressing a few buttons to administer insulin is a lot easier than setting up a pen for injection. For example, when out to eat at a restaurant where there are lots of small plates and different food selections it can be inconvenient to perform a pen injection every time food is put in front you, however, with a pump it is a lot easier to manage such a situation.

Despite the many advantages of the pump it is important for those contemplating moving onto one to consider if it is a preferable option over pen injections for themselves. An insulin pump must be worn almost all the time and it can be a nuisance constantly having something attached to your body. As a Diabetic friend of mine says, 'once on the pump you become 1% machine'. The pump can however be taken off for short periods of time such as when going for a swim or when showering, however, it has to be worn overnight and generally at all other times. In addition, pump users often get a lot of people asking 'what's that thing?' as, depending on where you wear it, it can stand out. Personally I take enjoyment in explaining to the uninformed what the pump is, what it is doing and why I wear it, and for the most part I find people are genuinely interested to learn more.

Insulin Administration Tips Summary

- Be mindful that most long-acting insulins have a slight dip in their action towards the end of their 12/24 hour cycle
- Use graphs showing insulin level against time for each insulin type and/or brand you used. Compare the graphs to identify specific times of the day where there may be more or less insulin acting in the body than desired and adjust your insulin regime accordingly
- For leaner individuals, pinch the skin at the injection site using your thumb and index finger and then inject into the raised skin fold. This keeps the needle within the area of subcutaneous fat
- Continually rotate injection sites to ensure one area is not being overused
- Again for leaner individuals, the abdomen and upper buttocks make the best injection sites, while employing the pinching technique
- When administering insulin to treat high BG levels, rub the injection site to get blood flowing in the area and thereby causing the insulin to act faster
- Always store insulin in the fridge at a stable temperature of approximately 4°C (39°F).

CHAPTER 3
DIET PLAN

Utilising Carbohydrate Counting

One of the most important skills to learn for improving your BG control is carbohydrate counting. In a nutshell, this is working out the amount of carbohydrate in grams (CHO/g) for every meal or snack you consume, and then using that number to work out how much rapid-acting insulin you require. Most Insulin-dependent Diabetics need approximately $1IU$ (1 unit of rapid-acting insulin) to cover 10-15g of carbohydrate. The math involved is fairly simple to implement once you get used to it but to provide context I will go through an example involving a typical carbohydrate source, in this case a serving of sweet potatoes.

Firstly, take the nutrition information for sweet potato that is provided in Figure 7. For 100g of sweet potatoes, there are 21g of carbohydrate. For someone that requires $1IU$ per 10g of carbohydrate, they would require $2IU$ for 100g of sweet potato (21 divided by 10 approximately equals 2, therefore 2*IU* is required).

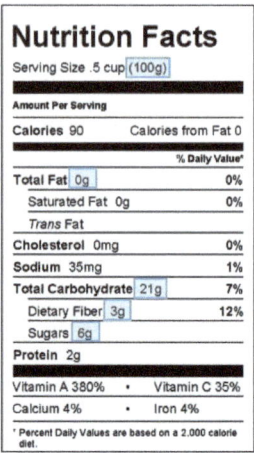

Figure 7 Example of extracting important information from a nutrition label. Shown here are the nutrition facts for 100g (total weight) of raw sweet potato.

Where carbohydrate counting becomes a bit trickier is when considering your insulin sensitivity at the time of eating. While it is a good starting point to use the same ratio of insulin to carbohydrate throughout the day, most Diabetics will find they need more or less insulin depending on the time of day, exercise performed that day or even due to more sporadic things such as stress level. While it is only ever possible to estimate your insulin requirements, I will provide some useful information to make your estimates as accurate as possible.

A common time of day where your insulin to carbohydrate ratio may increase is in the morning. As part of the waking up process, your body releases hormones which in turn stimulate the liver to release stored-up glucose. This is known in the Diabetic community as the 'dawn-phenomena'. If you use a pump, the best way to deal with this is to set an increase in your basal insulin rate to cover the time at which you've noticed your BG levels to be rising in the morning. I recommend setting the pump to increase the basal rate an hour before BG levels start to rise, and to decrease the long-acting rate back to normal an hour before BG levels start to go back to normal. This is due to the 'lag' effect of insulin action time as discussed in Chapter 2. However, for pen users, altering slow-acting (basal) insulin rates for short periods of time isn't an option, and in this case the best course of action is to increase your insulin to carbohydrate ratio instead. A good starting point for a Diabetic who requires say 1IU for every 15g carbohydrates throughout the day but is finding that their BG levels are high after breakfast, is to try 1IU to 10g carbohydrates (a 50% increase in insulin) to cover their breakfast and then continue at say 1IU to 15g carbohydrates for the rest of the day as normal. Naturally, this is a process requiring trial and error and it may take a number of adjustments to find what works best for you. With that said, it is important to slowly increase your insulin doses when doing so in order to avoid over-doing it and causing hypos.

You might find that like most people, some days you wake up not feeling hungry despite having been fasting for a long time during your sleep. This is due to the fact your liver releases glucose at a steady state while you sleep. This process provides the body with energy to repair overnight which is why Diabetics need long-acting insulin on board in order to deal with this released glucose.

Using the Glycemic Index to Better Match Food and Insulin

To take carbohydrate counting a step further, Diabetics can also account for the glycemic index (GI) of the various carbohydrate sources they consume. Each carbohydrate source has a different assigned GI ranging from 0 to 100 which essentially is a numerical value showing the amount of carbohydrates in the specific food that will turn into glucose and that will then enter the blood following consumption. In other words the GI of a food is the actual amount of carbohydrates you should be covering with insulin as this is the amount of insulin the body will actually require to process the food.

You may have noticed by now that some foods state a certain amount of carbohydrate content but when you dose insulin to match the carbohydrate content your BG levels don't behave as expected. Hopefully the information presented here will help you deal with this problem. Again for context I will provide an example of how to account for GI. Take the data provided in Table 2 for bananas. One large banana weighs 136g and has a net carbohydrate content of 27g (net carbohydrate equals total carbohydrate content minus the fiber content). As can be seen the GI of a banana is given as 52. This can be thought of as saying 52% of the carbohydrate content of the banana ends up as glucose in the blood and as such only 52% of the carbohydrate content needs to be covered by insulin. So, for 1 large banana, the carbohydrate content after accounting for the GI will be 14g of carbohydrates (27g multiplied by 0.52 (52%) which approximately equals 14g) which is also known as the glycemic load (GL). This means for an insulin-dependent Diabetic using a ratio of 1IU to 10g carbohydrates, 1.5IU will be required to cover the banana (14g divided by 10g approximately equals 1.5IU). Another consideration is that lower GI foods (GI 0-30) tend to contain more fiber content by weight than high GI foods (GI 70-100) and therefore digest slower.

This may seem like information overload, but once you gain sufficient practice in accounting for GI the process becomes much easier. To get started I recommend using Table 2 for quickly looking up the GI of various foods and for helping to account for GI in these foods. I should also add that once you start accounting for GI, you might find that your insulin to carbohydrate ratio increases. This is understandable as if you have not been previously accounting for GI you will have been overestimating the amount of carbohydrate in food sources which as a result underestimates your insulin to carbohydrate ratio.

One final consideration when carbohydrate counting is that the chosen cooking method can alter the GI of certain foods. Sticking with the example of sweet potato, you will find that the carbohydrate content changes depending on the method of cooking. If the sweet potato is oven cooked the carbohydrate content will stay the same as listed on the raw nutrition information, however, if the same quantity of sweet potato is boiled instead the carbohydrate content is lower despite using the exact same amount for each cooking method. In some cases the carbohydrate content can reduce by as much as half as what is listed on the raw nutrition information. The science behind why this happens is that boiling sweet potato doesn't separate the carbohydrate content fully from the fiber content of which it is bundled with in its raw state and as a result a relatively large amount of the carbohydrates contained within the sweet potato simply passes through the body, attached to fiber, without entering the blood stream as glucose.

Table 2 Glycemic Index and Glycemic Load of typical foods [6].

CHO Source	Glycemic Index	Serving Size	Net CHO	Glycemic Load
Pizza	30	2 slices (260g)	42	13
Low fat yogurt	33	1 cup (245g)	47	16
Apples	38	1 medium (138g)	16	6
Spaghetti	42	1 cup (140g)	38	16
Carrots	47	1 large (72g)	5	2
Oranges	48	1 medium (131g)	12	6
Bananas	52	1 large (136g)	27	14
Crisps	54	1 bag (35g)	16	9
Chocolate bar	55	1 bar (113g)	64	35
White rice	64	1 cup (186g)	52	33
Brown rice	55	1 cup (186g)	40	22
Oats	58	1 cup (234g)	21	12
Ice cream	61	1 cup (72g)	16	10
Macaroni and cheese	64	1 serving (166g)	47	30
Raisins	64	1 small box (43g)	32	20
White bread	70	1 slice (30g)	14	10
Brown bread	60	1 slice (30g)	12	7
Watermelon	72	1 cup (154g)	11	8
Popcorn	72	2 cups (16g)	10	7
Baked potato	85	1 medium (173g)	33	28
Boiled sweet potato	46	1 medium (173g)	30	14
Glucose	100	50g	50	50

The Low Carbohydrate Diet

The Low Carbohydrate Diet has become popular with Insulin-dependent Diabetics in recent years. The diet involves lowering your carbohydrate intake from the average for most people, which is approximately 300g of carbohydrates per day, to anything between 30 to 75g of net carbohydrates. When doing so it is important one increases their protein and fat content so that the overall daily calorie intake stays the same as is recommended for a person of their BMI. I should make clear that this is not the same as the Ketogenic Diet which involves cutting out carbohydrates altogether. While the Ketogenic Diet can be just as if not more successful in improving your BG control when compared to the Low Carbohydrate Diet, I personally find it to be unsustainable, which is not to say it won't work for others.

The major benefit of Low Carbohydrate Diets is that it stops big swings in BG levels that are common when eating high carbohydrate meals. Although most doctors will tell insulin-dependent Diabetics to eat what they like within reason so long as they cover it with the correct amount of insulin, this doesn't account for the fact that prescribed artificial insulin acts at a different rate to naturally produced insulin in non-diabetics. As previously mentioned, insulin can take a while to kick-in once injected and you may often find that your BG level rises way above the target range before the insulin pulls it back down to within target. These highs, while brief, can be damaging to the body in the long-run, however they can be easily mitigated by sticking to low carbohydrate meals.

When first starting a Low Carbohydrate Diet, it is common to feel tired and hungry but so long as total calorie intake is sufficient and the diet is stuck with, energy levels should return to normal after one to two weeks. A useful tip is to add one to two carbohydrate 're-load' meals per week to the diet plan. This involves every so often having a high carbohydrate meal that you enjoy which will help keep you happy and energized. A little tip I would add is to aim to have your carbohydrate re-load meals after exercise. This is because at this time your muscles are drained of glucose and much of the carbohydrates will be used to refuel the muscles instead of sitting stagnant in the blood stream, which helps prevent post-meal spikes in BG levels.

Another advantage of the Low Carbohydrate Diet is that it greatly reduces the amount of insulin needed each day. Preliminary studies have shown that excess insulin in the body can help fuel free radicals which are toxic byproducts of oxygen metabolism which in turn can cause significant damage to living cells and tissues in a process called oxidative stress.

Some further advice I can give you when trying out a Low Carbohydrate Diet is to avoid eating carbohydrates a few hours before going to bed. I've found this prevents storage of glucose in the liver which helps in preventing the dawn phenomena, where as previously discussed, the liver dumps glucose into the blood stream in the morning causing a BG spike.

Diet Considerations for Children with Diabetes

The majority of doctors discourage Low Carbohydrate Diets for patients below the age of 16. This is because it's believed carbohydrates play an important role in aiding cognitive development of growing children and teenagers. The same principles apply to pregnant women who suffer from Diabetes. In these cases consult your personal health professional before starting the diet to obtain the best course of action.

High Fat Meals

High fat meals, such as a carbohydrate re-load meal, require specific insulin regimes to properly cover their effects on BG levels. High fat meals can be defined as a meal with more than 20g of fat in it. The issue with high fat meals is that high fat consumption affects the body's digestive system in a way that reduces the potency of the injected insulin and at the same time slows down the rate at which glucose enters the blood from the stomach. A general way to account for this is to inject double the amount of insulin over a staggered period for time.

For pump users who can set 'square' or 'combo' bolus administrations, I recommend doubling the amount of insulin normally taken for the carbohydrate content in the food and administering it evenly over a two to three hour period of time (i.e. a squared bolus over two to three hours). Unfortunately this is not possible for pen users, however, a work around with pen injections is to also double the normal insulin requirement but inject 50% (of the doubled amount) immediately before eating and then the other 50% 1 hour after finishing the meal. By doing so the pen injected insulin will act similar to a square bolus administration by a pump user.

Example Meal Plan

Table 3 gives an example of a daily meal plan while following a Low Carbohydrate Diet for someone who requires 3000 calories of food per day. Generally, my own daily meal plan looks something like this.

Table 3 Example meal plan while following a Low Carbohydrate Diet Plan.

Meal	CHO sources	Net CHO	Protein source	Fat source
Breakfast	1 sachet of oats (28g)	17g	Scrambled egg whites	1/2 Avocado, 1 tablespoon of olive oil
Mid-morning snack			Plain beef jerky	Handful of almond nuts
Lunch	Whole wheat tortilla wrap (65g)	27g	Tuna with mayonnaise	1/2 Avocado, 1 tablespoon of olive oil
Mid-afternoon snack	1 Apple (138g)	16g		30g Dark chocolate
Dinner	Cauliflower rice (300g)	0g	Turkey with reduced sugar tomato sauce	High fat desert: 1 tablespoon of peanut butter, reduced sugar jelly, light whipped cream
Evening snack			Low carbohydrate protein shake	Handful of almond nuts

Insulin Off-setting Techniques

With basic understanding of GI values and the GI value of certain carbohydrate sources, an Insulin-dependent Diabetic can time their insulin injection so that it acts most efficiently for the carbohydrate being consumed. For the case of high GI carbohydrates (GI 70-100) we have already discussed that these tend to digest quickly. This means that if a person injects immediately before eating, their BG level will rise too high before the insulin pulls it back down, however if the person injects 15 minutes prior to eating the insulin action and BG rise will act much more accurately. This in turn prevents post-meal spikes. Vice versa, low GI carbohydrates (GI 0-30) are best covered by injecting 15 minutes post-eating due to the slow digestion of food. As for medium GI foods (GI 30-70), insulin should be injected immediately prior to eating.

Using off-setting techniques should be done with caution as it requires good understanding of how your BG levels react to different carbohydrates. Additionally, it can be risky to inject 15 minutes prior to eating carbohydrates as you may forget to eat the carbohydrate after injecting the insulin which could cause a hypo.

Diet Plan Tips Summary

- Use carbohydrate counting to best match insulin with consumed carbohydrates
- Always consider your insulin sensitivity at the time of eating
- Be mindful that during the waking up process, your body releases hormones which in turn stimulate the liver to release stored-up glucose, potentially causing BG level spikes
- Set up insulin increases/decreases an hour before noted BG level rises/falls, respectively, and increase/decrease back to normal an hour before BG level typically steady out
- When increasing insulin doses, do so slowly in order to avoid over-doing it and causing hypos
- Try to account for the GI of the various carbohydrate consumed in order to better match insulin doses with carbohydrate quantity
- Be mindful that different cooking methods can alter the GI of certain carbohydrate sources
- When on the Low Carbohydrate Diet stick to between 30-75g of net carbohydrate per day
- When on the Low Carbohydrate Diet it is important to increase protein and fat consumption so that your overall daily calorie intake stays the same as is recommended for a person of your BMI
- Add one to two carbohydrate re-load meals per week when on the Low Carbohydrate Diet to restore energy levels
- Aim to have carbohydrate re-load meals after exercise when your muscles are drained of glucose
- Avoid eating carbohydrates a few hours before going to bed to prevent storage of glucose in the liver which can subsequently cause a BG level spike in the morning

- When having high fat meals, you may need to inject double the amount of insulin over a staggered period for time
- Make use of insulin off-setting techniques to prevent BG level spikes.

CHAPTER 4
TREATING HYPOGLYCEMIC
ATTACKS

Suggested Treatments

Hypoglycemia, also known as low blood sugar, is when a person's BG level falls below the normal level. This can result in a variety of symptoms including clumsiness, trouble speaking, confusion, loss of consciousness, seizures or unfortunately even death. A feeling of hunger, sweating, shakiness and weakness can all also be present with symptoms generally appearing quickly. The diagnostic definition for Diabetics is a BG level below 3.9mmol/L (70mg/dL) [7].

The recommended treatment for hypos is usually 10 to 20g of rapid-acting carbohydrate (glucose) immediately upon noticing the hypo. However, you may often find that this recommended amount raises BG levels too much or too little. This is due to a number of factors, the main ones being the person's body weight and the severity of the hypo. Please note that the section immediately following this one gives information on how to calculate the correct amount of rapid-acting carbohydrate to consume in order to treat hypos while taking into account body weight and hypo severity.

The main choice of hypo treatment is sugar tablets with the main brand being dextrose, however, I recommend using liquid fast-acting carbohydrates such as pure orange juice or full-sugar soft drinks as the glucose in these gets to action quicker as there is no 'breaking down' phase in the digestive track. Taking the example of orange juice, it has approximately 10g of sugar per 100ml meaning a standard small carton (normally 200ml in content) is perfect for treating a hypo. Another tip while on the subject of treating hypos is to always ensure your BG monitor kit is clean. During the frantic dash of treating a hypo it is easy to get some sugar on your kit which can give false high readings the next time you use it. Of course the same applies to making sure your hands are clean before testing.

Following treatment of a hypo, once BG levels have returned to a safe range, it is important to consider how much insulin is on board. If there is still a lot of insulin in your system it is likely you may go back into a hypo range. This is easier to track for pump users, so I would recommend pen users keep a diary record of their insulin doses and their action times which can then be easily consulted following a hypo. In addition, to be extra conservative I like to reduce my rapid-acting insulin dose by half of what it would normally be for meals that soon follow a hypo episode. This helps to avoid a repeat episode and I can always correct back down an hour after the meal if my BG levels go too high due to this. For pump users I would also recommend putting on a temporary basal reduction of 20% for three to four hours, again just to be on the safe side.

This final piece of advice is not directly for Diabetics but for Diabetics to pass on to their close friends, families and colleagues that may have to treat your hypo if you are unable to do so yourself. When a Diabetic is unconscious they will not be able to swallow fast-acting carbohydrate however it can be rubbed onto the Diabetic's gums. This works because glucose can enter the bloodstream through the small vessels close to the surface of the gums and in certain scenarios it may be the only treatment option. This is best done with glucose gel but if the only available treatment is sugar tablets, these can be crushed up or even chewed up by someone (putting hygiene concerns aside for a moment) if necessary and placed onto the gums of the Diabetic.

Carbohydrate Requirements for Treating Hypoglycemic Attacks

Table 4 on the following page shows the different amounts of fast-acting carbohydrates needed to correct low BG levels for varying bodyweights. It can be seen that those of lower body weight require less fast-acting glucose while those of higher body weight require more. The reason for this is quite intuitive in that a lower body-weight person generally has less blood in their body which means that the fast-acting glucose needs to be 'mixed' with the blood to bring BG levels into a safe range. To illustrate this further, imagine an 80kg person is having a hypo attack with a BG reading at 3.0mmol/L. This person would want to raise their BG level to a safe range of say 5.6mmol/L, so going off of Table 4, the person would need approximately 12g of fast-acting glucose (5.6mmol/L minus 3.0mmol/L equals 2.6mmol/L, therefore 2.6mmol/L divided by 0.22mmol/L/g which equals approximately 12g of fast-acting glucose, is required). Personally, I believe it is always best to be conservative so in this case I would recommend rounding up to 15g of fast-acting carbohydrate to treat the hypo.

Table 4 Increase in blood glucose level upon consumption of 1g of glucose in relation to the bodyweight of an individual [8].

Body Weight (kg)	Blood Glucose Level Increase After Consuming 1g of Glucose (mmol/L/g)
16	1.11
32	0.56
48	0.39
64	0.28
80	0.22
95	0.18
111	0.17
128	0.14
143	0.12

Hypo Awareness

Most Diabetics who have lived with the disease for many years will know that over time the ability to detect a hypo as it is coming on starts to fade with severity and frequency of hypos. This is simply because the brain adapts to functioning at a lower BG level and loses the ability to physically signal the body via the central nervous system that a hypo is occurring. Specifically, warning signs such as shaky hands and dizziness only start to arise at BG levels lower than would be preferred. The technical term for this is 'inhibited hypo awareness'.

Fortunately Diabetics who suffer from inhibited hypo awareness can restore their hypo awareness and the brains sensitivity in terms of reacting to hypos. This is done through better Diabetes control with the aim of reducing the frequency and severity of hypos that the Diabetic experiences. By doing so, this makes the event of a hypo more of a 'shock' to the brain again causing it to respond proficiently. My advice for Diabetics who suffer from repeated hypo attacks with low hypo awareness is to run your BG level slightly higher than the standard target range i.e. instead of 4.0mmol/L to 7.5mmol/L aim towards 5.0mmol/L to 9.0mmol/L. While this is not an ideal long term management strategy it should help towards raising hypo awareness. Following this, once hypo awareness has returned, the individual should go back to using the standard BG target range, this time being more vigilant of what was causing the hypos initially and adjusting their management and/or lifestyle accordingly to prevent them.

Treating Hypoglycemic Attacks Tips Summary

- Calculate the correct amount of rapid-acting carbohydrate you need to consume in order to treat hypos while taking into account your body weight and hypo severity
- It is better to use liquid fast-acting carbohydrates such as pure orange juice or full-sugar soft drinks as the glucose in these gets to action quicker than solid alternatives e.g. sugar tablets
- Always ensure your BG monitor kit and hands are clean before testing
- Following treatment of a hypo, once BG levels have returned to a safe range, consider how much insulin you have on board. If there is still a lot of insulin in your system it is likely you may go back into hypo range
- Following treatment of a hypo, reduce your rapid-acting insulin dose by half of what it would normally be for meals that soon follow a the hypo episode
- Teach family members and friends how to treat you if you are having a hypo in cases where you can't do so yourself
- Be mindful that the ability to detect a hypo as it is arising starts to fade with severity and frequency of hypos
- For Diabetics who suffer from repeated hypo attacks with low hypo awareness, it is useful to run your BG level slightly higher than the standard target range, until sensitivity has returned.

CHAPTER 5
PHYSICAL ACTIVITY

Monitoring Blood Glucose around Physical Activity

When engaging in physical activity a Diabetic should test their BG level at the following times:

- 15 minutes prior to starting physical activity
- Every 15 to 30 minutes during physical activity
- Immediately after physical activity has ended.

Of course the above requirements can vary significantly depending on the type and intensity of exercise being performed, however, this should serve as a good starting point for anyone unsure about managing their Diabetes around exercise.

For CGM users, I would recommend reverting back to your finger-stick monitor when testing BG levels around exercise. This is because the longer delay time of the CGM, as previously discussed, is more of an issue during times of rapidly changing BG levels, as is often the case when exercising. As such a finger-stick monitor is more effective for keeping BG levels in check around exercise.

Diabetic treatment items needed during exercise do not differ greatly from what a Diabetic should be carrying at all times. However, just to provide a comprehensive list I will note everything I personally take with me when exercising:

- Fast acting glucose – small carton of pure orange juice
- Backup fast acting glucose – Dextrose tablets
- Snacks to maintain BG levels if need be – two cereal bars
- Backup insulin pens (in case my insulin pump fails)
- Backup finger-stick BG monitor and testing strips (in case my primary BG monitor fails)
- Medical ID band around my wrist in case of an emergency.

As you can see I carry an extensive amount of Diabetes paraphernalia around with me, however you would be surprised just how often the backup items come in handy. I recommend ensuring you have all the items listed above and do your best to carry them around as often as possible. Carrying everything in a small pouch bag can make life a little easier.

A final point I will make is that the aforementioned tips also apply to many physical activities, not just sport. For example, activities such as cleaning the house, food and clothes shopping, and packing for say going on a trip are all surprisingly physically demanding. Activities such as those listed can have a pronounced effect on BG levels. Naturally, the effect on BG levels if highly dependent on the type and length of activity but as a rule of thumb you should treat any activity that you feel may affect your BG levels the same as you would for exercising.

Insulin Requirements around Physical Activity

For Diabetics who are also athletes, it is important to note that carbohydrates consumption (as mentioned in Chapter 3) can be very beneficial in terms of body recovery and performance, as previously touched on when discussing carbohydrate 're-load' meals. In addition, you will find that after intense workouts, the muscles are starved of glucose. This often means that the insulin dosage for post-workout meals has to be reduced as the body needs less of it to process the incoming glucose. This occurs due to Insulin sensitivity increasing during and after exercise meaning that muscle cells are better able to use any available insulin to take up glucose during this time. Interestingly, it is believed that during exercise, when muscles contract, the cells within the muscles are able to take up glucose and use it for energy whether insulin is available or not [9].

To give you a better idea of how to go about dosing insulin before, during and after workouts, I will give my regime around a one hour swimming training session. Note that some of these points involve using an insulin pump; however, most of it applies to pen injections as well:

- 1.5 hours prior to starting session – reduce basal rate by 100% (i.e. no basal insulin being administered at all)
- Maintain 100% reduced basal rate during session (I remove my pump while swimming)
- Immediately post-session – put pump back on and set a reduced basal rate of 30% for five hours (i.e. basal rate set to 70% of normal value for five hours)
- Post-session meal – only administer half of my normal insulin dose for the meal I am having.

Diabetic Athletes

For inspiration, a list of notable Diabetic athletes and teams is provided hear. All of the individuals mentioned here have overcome the obstacles presented by Diabetes and achieved success at an elite sporting level. While this may be of more interest to Diabetic athletes reading this book, I hope the stories of these people provide motivation for thriving in life despite the limitations of Diabetes.

Team Novo Nordisk

Team Novo Nordisk is an all-Diabetes professional cycling team that competes against some of the best non-Diabetic athletes in the world in both male and female cycling competitions. The team is the first of its kind and acts as a great ambassador to Diabetic athletes who don't want to let their disease hold them back.

Team Novo Nordisk has a very inclusive attitude and encourages all interested Diabetics to get involved. I highly recommend checking out their official website which provides some very insightful tips into managing Diabetes around exercise along with the personal stories of each individual rider on the team.
(www.teamnovonordisk.com)

Gary Hall Jr

Gary Hall Jr. is a former competitive swimmer and is one of the most successful swimmers of the United States swim team in its history. He won ten Olympic medals, five of which were gold, between 1996 and 2004 while specializing in freestyle sprint events. Amazingly he achieved much of his success while suffering from Type 1 Diabetes.

In 2012 Hall was inducted into the United States

Olympic Hall of Fame. Again, I encourage reading more into his life and career along with interviews he has given regarding how he best manages the disease.

Sir Steve Redgrave

Sir Steve Redgrave is a retired rower who is widely considered to be one of Britain's greatest ever Olympians in addition to being one of the most decorated Olympians of all time. Amazingly, Redgrave won gold medals at five consecutive games between 1984 and 2000 despite being diagnosed with Type 2 Diabetes in 1997.

Following his diagnosis, Redgrave was put on a low-sugar diet, however as a high performing athlete he felt this left his energy levels too low and as such changed back to a high-calorie diet. While this slightly contradicts the sentiment of Low Carbohydrate Dieting, it should be noted that intense daily exercise, especially at level required for an Olympic athlete, requires a person to have a large carbohydrate intake due to carbohydrates being an efficient source of energy.

Despite initial concerns regarding achieving the goals he set out before his diagnosis, Redgrave overcame the obstacles of the disease to achieve even more success. He notes this was in part thanks to advice from medical professionals that gave him the confidence to continue rowing.

Physical Activity Tips Summary

- Test BG level 15 minutes prior to starting physical activity
- Test BG level every 15 to 30 minutes during physical activity
- Test BG level immediately after physical activity has ended
- For CGM users, it is a good idea to use your finger-stick monitor when testing BG levels around exercise due to the shorter lag time of the reading
- Insure you carry all of the recommended Diabetic treatment items needed during exercise
- Carrying everything in a small pouch bag can be convenient
- Be mindful that activities such as cleaning the house, food and clothes shopping, and packing for say going on a trip can have a pronounced effect on BG levels
- In most cases, insulin dosage for post-workout meals has to be reduced as the body needs less of it to process the incoming glucose.

CHAPTER 6
SOCIAL LIFE

Going Out to Eat

Prior to heading out to eat it's always a good idea to ensure you have all treatment items you may possibly need. This includes, but is not limited to, sufficient insulin supplies, testing strips, a primary glucose monitor, a backup glucose monitor, snacks and sufficient hypo treatment. All of this adds up to a lot of things to carry around with you and it can be quite a nuisance when you're just trying to enjoy yourself while out to eat. I recommend getting a big enough pouch bag or purse that can hold all these things and then keep it on you at all times while out.

As most Diabetics know, when you fancy a soft drink it is preferable to go with the diet option due to the zero-sugar content, unless you're having a hypo of course. However, often when you order a soft drink it comes in a glass instead of the original can or bottle. There have been a couple of times where I've ordered a diet soft drink but ended up with the non-diet alternative in a glass.

Unfortunately, I'm awful at distinguishing between diet and non-diet soft-drink by taste and as such in these instances my BG levels sky-rocketed unbeknown to me. Nowadays, I always ask for the drink to come in the original bottle to confirm it is what I intended to order or if this is not possible I will explain my situation to the person serving me to ensure they don't make a mistake.

Another issue that can arise while going out to eat is having no idea how much carbohydrate is in the meals you've ordered. The best solution for this is to download a 'carb counting' app onto your phone. The one I use is called 'Carbs & Cals' which not only provides the carbohydrate content of a variety of foods but also gives a breakdown for different portion sizes. I'm sure there are many different apps to choose from so it's probably best to look around and find the one that works well for you.

Once you know the amount of carbohydrates you're having, then comes the time to administer you're insulin in front of everyone. A few Diabetics I have spoken to have told me they often feel hesitant about doing this in front of others, especially those they don't know that well. My advice would be to just go for it! It's a real inconvenience for you having to do this in the first place and anyone you're eating with should be willing to accommodate your treatment and not ask you something silly like 'could you do that in the bathroom instead?' In my experience, whenever someone sees me testing my BG levels or administering insulin and they didn't realise I was Diabetic they normally are curious to find out more about it and this leads to an enjoyable conversion.

One final tip would be to always wait until your food is served and right in front of you before administering your insulin. As we all know, food often arrives late and the portion sizes are often different than what was expected when ordering so naturally it is a bad idea to try and guess how much insulin is needed before actually seeing the food in front of you. As a side note, always try to inject insulin before, not after, meals, unless you know the carbohydrate source is going to digest very slowly, as previously discussed. The reason for this goes back to the delayed action of insulin and trying to time BG rise with insulin action.

Nights Out

When heading on a night out it is always a good idea to give spare hypo treatment to one of the members of your group just in case you have a hypo that for whatever reason you can't treat yourself.

If you're on a night out and plan on drinking alcohol I would advise sticking to beer, red wine or spirits (mixed with diet soft-drinks if desired). The reason for this is that all of these have a very low effect on your BG levels. That may seem to be a counter-intuitive statement as beer and red wine are often classed as 'high-calorie', however much of the carbohydrates that makes up the calorie content in these drinks has been refined in such a way that once it enters the body it doesn't actually enter the bloodstream and as such doesn't raise BG levels.

For me personally, I don't need to take any insulin when having these aforementioned drinks. However, that is not to say these drinks have absolutely no impact on your BG levels, in fact all alcohol does and does so to varying degrees. Even though many alcoholic drinks don't initially raise BG levels and don't require insulin administration, the effects of alcohol on the liver can lower insulin requirements for Diabetics after having been consumed. Essentially, after drinking the liver becomes pre-occupied by having to process the alcohol and as such stops releasing the steady flow of glucose it would be releasing otherwise. This means that a Diabetic will need to decrease their long-acting (basal) insulin rate for a period of time following consumption of alcohol. There is no rule of thumb for this as the amount by which the long-acting rate needs to be decreased is highly dependent on the amount and type of alcohol consumed. However, to provide more clarity, personally for me, after having drank say two pints of beer, I will decrease my basal rate by 30% for six hours to match the time in which my liver has to deal with the alcohol. Again, this may not work for everyone and it certainly requires some trial and error to find what works best for you.

One final point I will make is to always do your best to inform everyone in your group about your condition. You never know when you may need their help.

Social Life Tips Summary

- When going out for social events, always bring sufficient insulin supplies, testing strips, a primary glucose monitor, a backup glucose monitor, snacks and sufficient hypo treatment
- When ordering soft-drinks, always ask for the drink to come in the original bottle to confirm it is what you intended to order
- Download a carb counting app onto your phone
- Always wait until your food is served and right in front of you before administering your insulin
- Give spare hypo treatment to one of the members of your group when out for a social event
- Stick to beer, red wine or spirits (mixed with diet soft-drinks if desired) as these tend not to raise your BG level
- Be mindful that the effects of alcohol on the liver can lower insulin requirements for Diabetics after having been consumed
- Depending on quantity of alcohol consumed you may need to decrease your long-acting insulin rate for a period of time following consumption
- Always do your best to inform everyone in your group about your condition.

CHAPTER 7
TRAVELLING

Packing Your Diabetes Supplies

Leaving plenty of packing time prior to travelling for a holiday, business trip or for any other travel reason is especially important for Diabetics. When going abroad, your access to health care is limited so sufficient medical supplies should be taken with you from home which should include backup items in case you lose anything while away from home.

I once had a situation where I was on holiday in Spain and my glucose meter was stolen (I assume someone mistook the pouch that contained the meter for a wallet or a purse). Luckily I had a backup meter which I was able to use, however, I only had a limited number of testing strips for this backup meter. I went around all the pharmacies at the resort to try and buy more testing strips only to find that the brand of strips my meter used was not sold in Spain! By sheer luck one of the receptionists that worked at the hotel I was staying at was a Type 1 Diabetic too and she very kindly gave me a spare meter with plenty of testing strips. In this case I was fortunate, but as you can imagine in more remote areas of the world such situations could be much more serious and quickly become life-threatening. The lesson of this story is always bring spare supplies and bring enough to last you for the entirety of the trip.

In terms of travelling to your destination I recommend buying 'cool bags' to store your insulin while on the move. This keeps the insulin cool meaning you don't have to worry about it over-heating and spoiling. These can be easily bought online. The ones I like to use are called FRIO bags.

Insulin maintains its potency at room temperature for approximately a month before losing its effectiveness, as such putting it into cool bags while travelling isn't absolutely necessary, however, when it's packed away it can be exposed to a wide range of temperatures so I personally feel it's always best to take the precaution of putting it into a cool bag.

Moving onto carrying your insulin on flights, it is best to take all of your insulin with you into the plane cabin i.e. don't put it into the hold inside your suitcase. The temperature is significantly lower in the hold hence your insulin could be effected. Additionally, you may want to give half of your supplies to someone travelling with you in case you lose your carry-on bag containing your insulin.

Going through Airport Security

As previously mentioned a lot of your Diabetic supplies need to be carried on you which means taking them through airport security. I advise getting a signed doctors letter from either your Doctor or the Diabetic clinic you attend. Personally, I've never had to show my Doctor's letter to anyone but it's still a good idea to keep it on you, just in case. Normally I have insulin, needles and my insulin pump on me while I go through airport security. The insulin and needles never cause a problem, however, my insulin pump can't be put through the X-ray machine in case it gets damaged. As such I have to wear it through the body scanner and every time it triggers the machine. At this point I just tell the staff that I'm wearing an insulin pump which doesn't cause any issues as most security personnel have seen one before. The security personnel do however 'swab' the pump to check it (this is completely safe in terms of pump care) and occasionally I may have to go through a second body scanner, again without removing the pump. Note that some insulin pump manufacturers specify their pumps can't go through body scanners in addition to x-ray machines. Is this is this case it is important to inform the airport security staff and make sure you follow the manufacturer's instructions. All in all there are not too many issues when going through airport security except for the fact the process takes a bit longer than it would for a non-Diabetic.

It is also important to bring plenty of snacks and fast-acting glucose with you before entering an airport. As I am sure you are well aware, it is common to go long periods of time waiting in lines and at airport gates where you don't have access to shops to buy snacks. As such it is wise to stock up on these so that you always have them if needed.

Time Zone Changes

When travelling to different time zones it can be tricky to adjust your insulin regime to match your new schedule. If you are only spending a short length of time in a different time zone (i.e. a weekend) or if the time is only changing by an hour or two I personally wouldn't bother adjusting my regime, however, if you're away for a long time and the time is significantly different to your local time you will need to adjust things. Ideally, only your long-acting insulin injecting times need to change and it is best to do this incrementally each day. For example, if the new time zone is five hours behind your normal time zone, you should move your injection time back an hour every day for five days at which point you will be set up correctly for the new time zone. Try to avoid jumping your long-acting injection time straight to those of the new time zone as this will cause 'stacking' of the amount of insulin in the body which could lead to hypos.

In addition, your insulin quantity requirements may need to be altered depending on the type of trip your taking. If you are going on an action packed holiday I'd advise lowering the amount of insulin you take as the higher activity level will lead to the body requiring less insulin. Conversely, if you normally lead an active lifestyle and you plan on having a well-deserved relaxing holiday with plenty of good food I'd recommend increasing your insulin dosage.

It should also be noted that while the body adjusts to a new time zone it is important to test regularly to make sure the BG levels are in check as this is a time where they can be especially erratic. Finally, I should once again state this is not an exact science and you shouldn't be deterred if you don't get it right the first time as it certainly will take some practice to get right.

Travelling Tips Summary

- Always bring spare supplies on trips and bring enough to last you for the entirety of the trip
- Consider buying cool bags to store your insulin while you are travelling
- Always take all of your insulin with you into the plane cabin
- Give half of your treatment supplies to someone travelling with you when flying, in case you lose your carry-on bag containing them
- Get a signed doctors letter from either your Doctor or the Diabetic clinic in case you need to show it when going through airport security
- Be mindful that some insulin pumps can't go through body scanners or x-ray machines
- Bring plenty of snacks and fast-acting glucose with you when going through an airport
- If you're going to be away from home for a long time and the destination time is significantly different to your local time you will need to adjust your insulin regime
- Adjust insulin incrementally each day, if required
- Insulin dosage requirements, in addition to administration times, may need to be altered depending on the type of trip your taking
- While your body adjusts to a new time zone it is important to test regularly to make sure your BG level is in check as this is a time where they can be especially erratic.

CHAPTER 8
PRESCRIPTIONS

Requesting Different and New Treatments from Your Doctor

With the ever changing nature of the treatment available to Diabetics I recommend you keep on top of Diabetic care advancements so that you receive the best treatment available to you. This can be off putting as it requires going through the process of regularly setting up a new prescription with your doctor, however in most clinics I've been registered at, there are systems in place to make such requests easier. Normally you won't have to book an appointment and you can just simply call up the clinic to request a change of prescription or even show up at the clinic to fill out a quick form at reception.

In some cases, insurance companies and National Health Services aren't willing to provide new treatment due to budget constraints. If you feel you really need an item that is not provided (this is often the case with CGM sensors, although more recently more and more health services are starting to provide these) I recommend speaking with your doctor or even contacting the relevant funding body to explain why you need the specific item. Often an exception can be made for you if you provide a good reason for why you need a different or new treatment. In my experience it has often been a case of 'you don't ask you don't get' when it comes to getting non-standard treatment items. Additionally, do your own research into new products on the market that may be of benefit to you as it is unlikely your health service will inform you of absolutely everything that is available, especially if the items can't be covered by their budget.

On a more optimistic note I should add that most National Health Services, specifically the UK NHS which I use, do generally provide great treatment for Diabetics. This can be clearly seen when comparing modern day treatment to what it was thirty or so years ago. In most cases, the standard treatment provided is sufficient for enabling Diabetics to live long and healthy lives.

Future Treatments

It is very common to see headlines in the news regarding 'cures' and 'breakthrough treatments' for Diabetics. While it is encouraging to see this, often the proposed treatment never comes to fruition and drops off the radar completely. The reason for this is two-fold.

Firstly, many news platforms like to sensationalise health stories and secondly clinical trials are incredibly tedious. Focusing on the second point, when a new treatment or drug is produced it has to go through a long trial process where it is used on animals and human test groups in order to fully assess the safety and effectiveness of the item. In some cases this can be as long 10 years of testing which may seem excessive but is important to establish the long term effects of the treatment prior to releasing for wide scale use. This means that many of the headlining drugs and treatments you read about in the news are actually still in trial phase, many of which may go on to eventually fail at trial phase before release to the public is possible.

Unfortunately all us Diabetics can do is just be patient. We can however take comfort in the fact that there are a great number of research teams made up of very talented people trying to find a range of different ways to help Diabetics.

In terms of the most likely treatments that will be available in the near future the most exciting is the 'Closed-Loop System. Here, an insulin pump like machine will be attached to a Diabetic's body which not only delivers insulin but also continuously tests BG levels and administers insulin accordingly meaning there is no user input required. As you can imagine, this would make the life of Diabetic much easier and as such is definitely a space to watch. Another item that looks like it will be released in the near future is Skin-Patch BG monitors. Essentially this a small plaster-like patch that sits on the skin and remotely monitors BG levels through perspiration. Such a device would remove the need for the more invasive finger-stick and CGM monitoring.

A more complex treatment which is occasionally performed but still requires a lot of improvement is a pancreas transplant. Here a healthy pancreas is transplanted into a Type 1 Diabetic patient, replacing the unhealthy pancreas. Following the transplant the patient takes immuno-suppressant drugs to prevent the immune system from destroying cells in the new pancreas. While this sounds great in theory, the problem is that it requires a very invasive procedure which carries its own risks and additionally the immuno-suppressant treatment is required indefinitely following the transplant meaning the Diabetic still requires daily treatment. Personally I don't see this method of treatment becoming wide-scale in the future unless the limitations can be somehow alleviated. None-the-less, it is certainly interesting to think about.

As a closing point to this section and this eBook as a whole I would like to mention that the future looks increasingly bright for all types of Diabetics. As mentioned there are many potential treatments in the pipeline that if successful at trial will significantly improve our quality of life. In addition there is research being done into creating vaccine treatments that can be given to people who are genetically predisposed to develop Diabetes prior to them actually developing the illness so that it never arises, much like any other vaccination shot. Finally, while I can't make any sweeping statements about when Diabetes will likely be cured, indeed if it ever actually will be, I am quick to state that when I look back at the development of insulin treatment in the early 20th century and compare it to what is currently available it can be seem that exponential advancement has been made. If this trend of progress continues, it seems reasonable to think the disease will be cured or at the very least become nothing but a minor inconvenience to all those living with it.

Prescription Tips Summary

- Keep on top of Diabetic care advancements so that you receive the best treatment available to you
- If certain treatment options are not available on your insurance policy or National Health Service prescription, try speaking with your doctor or even contacting the relevant funding body to explain why you need the specific item. Often an exception can be made.

REFERENCES

[1] A. Basu *et al.*, "Time Lag of Glucose From Intravascular to Interstitial Compartment in Humans," *Diabetes,* vol. 62, pp. 4083-4087, 2013.

[2] T. Bailey, B. W. Bode, M. P. Christiansen, L. J. Klaff, and S. Alva, "The Performance and Usability of a Factory-Calibrated Flash Glucose Monitoring System," *Diabetes Technology & Therapeutics,* vol. 17, no. 11, pp. 787-794, 2015.

[3] International Organization for Standardization, "In vitro diagnostic test systems–requirements for blood-glucose monitoring systems for self-testing in managing diabetes mellitus," in "ISO report 15197," International Organization for Standardization, Geneva, Switzerland, 2003.

[4] J. S. Freeman, "Insulin Analog Therapy: Improving the Match With Physiologic Insulin Secretion," *The Journal of the American Osteopathic Association,* vol. 109, no. 1, pp. 26-36, 2009.

[5] E. Toschi, "Safe and effective use of insulin requires proper storage," *Harvard Health Publishing,* 2018.

[6] The University of Sydney. Glycemic Index [Online] Available: www.glycemicindex.com

[7] National Institute of Diabetes and Digestive and Kidney Diseases. Hypoglycemia

[8] R. K. Bernstein, *Dr. Bernstein's Diabetes Solution: The Complete Guide to Achieving Normal Blood Sugars,* 4 ed. Little, Brown Spark, 2011.

[9] American Diabetes Association. Blood Glucose and Exercise [Online] Available: www.diabetes.org/food-and-fitness/fitness/get-started-safely/blood-glucose-control-and-exercise.html

ABOUT THE AUTHOR

I am in unique situation where I am both a researcher into the biological effects of diabetes on the human body and a sufferer of Type 1 Diabetes.

At the age 20, the better part of a decade ago, I was diagnosed with Type 1 Diabetes. At the time, it was a bitter pill to swallow. I was just heading into the prime of my life; I was a competitive swimmer and right in the middle of my undergraduate studies, just starting to pave the path of my future life. Like most people diagnosed with diabetes my mindset drastically changed post-diagnosis. I recall being very concerned about the limitations the disease may set upon me and what aspects of my lifestyle would be permanently impacted.

Despite my initial feeling of anguish, I persevered and in the following years after my diagnosis, I decided to immerse myself in the literature surrounding diabetes to find the best solutions for tackling it. I learnt as much as could about diabetes management and continually sought ways to improve my control. To this day, the desire to improve my situation remains, which over time has proven very useful in terms of mitigating the negative effects of the disease. Moving on from my initial diagnosis, I continued to train as a competitive swimmer, I obtained a first class undergraduate degree from the University of Edinburgh in Structural Engineering and obtained my Masters degree from Imperial College London with a specific research focus in Bioengineering. At present, I am a member of a research team at McGill University in Montreal, Canada, looking into biomechanical degradation on implant design relating to a number of bodily ailments, one of which being diabetes.

At the time of writing, I have reached an HbA1c level of 5.8% whilst minimizing the number of hypoglycemic attacks I have to less than one a month. My HbA1c level puts my control just above the range of a non-Diabetic, something I'm very proud of. My hope is that with this eBook, you can take my knowledge, combine it with your own, and put it towards improving your HbA1c and diabetes control as a whole and match what I've done or hopefully surpass it.

S. H. McLennan

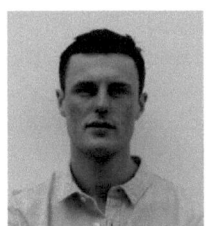

www.ingramcontent.com/pod-product-compliance
Lightning Source LLC
Chambersburg PA
CBHW040906180526
45159CB00010BA/2950